Essentials for Organic Homemade Skincare Routine on a budget for a perfect skin

A step by step guide DIY on production and daily usage of home made organic skincare products.

Schola Marshall

Chapter 1

Discover Your Skin Type

Your skin is as unique as you are, and understanding its individual needs is essential for achieving healthy, radiant, and glowing skin. Whether your skin is oily, dry, combination, or sensitive, knowing your skin type is the first step towards developing an effective skincare routine that addresses your specific concerns. In this guide, we'll explore the different skin types and how to identify yours, so you can choose the best skincare products for your skin's needs.

Identifying Your Skin Type:

1. Oily Skin:

- Characteristics: Oily skin is prone to excess sebum production, resulting in a shiny or greasy appearance, enlarged pores, and a tendency to develop acne or blemishes.

- How to Identify: If your skin feels greasy or looks shiny throughout the day, especially in the T-zone (forehead, nose, and chin), you likely have oily skin.

- Skincare Tips: Look for oil-free or non-comedogenic products that help control excess oil and minimize the appearance of pores without stripping the skin's natural moisture.

2. Dry Skin:

- Characteristics: Dry skin lacks moisture and often feels tight, rough, or flaky. It may appear dull, irritated, or prone to fine lines and wrinkles.

- How to Identify: If your skin feels tight or appears flaky, especially after cleansing or in harsh weather conditions, you likely have dry skin.

- Skincare Tips: Opt for hydrating and nourishing products that replenish moisture, strengthen the skin barrier, and soothe dryness and irritation. Look for ingredients like hyaluronic acid, glycerin, and ceramides.

3. Combination Skin:

- Characteristics: Combination skin features a mix of oily and dry areas, with an oily T-zone and drier cheeks or perimeter of the face.
- How to Identify: If your forehead, nose, and chin are oily, while your cheeks feel normal or dry, you likely have combination skin.
- Skincare Tips: Use products designed for combination skin that balance oil production in the T-zone while providing hydration and moisture to drier areas. Consider using different products for different areas of the face as needed.

4. Sensitive Skin:
- Characteristics: Sensitive skin is prone to irritation, redness, and inflammation in response to various triggers, such as harsh ingredients, environmental factors, or changes in weather.
- How to Identify: If your skin frequently reacts to skincare products, environmental factors, or changes in temperature, you likely have sensitive skin.

- Skincare Tips: Choose gentle, fragrance-free, and hypoallergenic products specifically formulated for sensitive skin. Avoid harsh ingredients like alcohol, fragrances, and sulfates that may cause irritation or exacerbate sensitivity.

Knowing your skin type is the foundation of a successful skincare routine tailored to your individual needs. By identifying your skin type and choosing products formulated to address its specific concerns, you can achieve healthier, more radiant skin. Remember to listen to your skin's needs, observe how it responds to different products, and adjust your skincare routine accordingly for optimal results. With the right knowledge and products, you can unlock the secrets to beautiful, glowing skin at any age.

Chapter 2

Getting Started

Embarking on an organic homemade skincare routine is a wonderful way to nourish your skin with natural ingredients while avoiding harsh chemicals and additives. By harnessing the power of nature's bounty, you can create effective skincare products tailored to your skin's unique needs. In this guide, we'll explore the essential ingredients, tools, and tips you need to start your journey to radiant, healthy skin with an organic homemade skincare routine.

1. Natural Ingredients:

- Essential Oils: Choose high-quality, organic essential oils such as lavender, tea tree, rosehip, or frankincense for their therapeutic benefits and skin-nourishing properties.

- Carrier Oils: Opt for cold-pressed, organic carrier oils like jojoba, argan, coconut, or almond oil to provide hydration, nourishment, and moisture to the skin.

- Herbs and Botanicals: Incorporate dried herbs and botanicals such as chamomile, calendula, rose petals, or green tea for their antioxidant, anti-inflammatory, and soothing properties.

2. Basic Ingredients:

- Raw Honey: A natural humectant and antibacterial agent, raw honey helps moisturize, soothe, and clarify the skin while promoting healing and regeneration.

- Aloe Vera Gel: Known for its soothing and hydrating properties, aloe vera gel helps calm inflammation, reduce redness, and promote skin healing.

- Shea Butter or Cocoa Butter: Rich in vitamins and fatty acids, shea butter and cocoa butter provide intense hydration, nourishment, and protection for dry or sensitive skin.

3. Tools and Equipment:

- Mixing Bowls and Spoons: Use glass or stainless steel mixing bowls and spoons to prepare your skincare formulations, as they are non-reactive and easy to clean.

- Storage Containers: Choose dark glass containers or jars with airtight lids to store your homemade skincare products and protect them from light and air exposure.

- Blender or Food Processor: For recipes that require blending or emulsifying ingredients, a blender or food processor can help achieve a smooth and uniform texture.

4. Recipe Books and Resources:

- Invest in recipe books, online resources, or skincare workshops that provide inspiration, guidance, and recipes for creating homemade skincare products.

- Experiment with different formulations, ingredients, and techniques to find what works best for your skin type and preferences.

5. Safety Precautions:

- Patch Test: Always perform a patch test before using a new skincare product to check for any allergic reactions or sensitivities.

- Cleanliness: Ensure that your hands, tools, and containers are clean and sanitized to prevent contamination and bacterial growth in your skincare products.

- Storage: Store your homemade skincare products in a cool, dry place away from direct sunlight to maintain their freshness and efficacy.

Conclusion:

Starting an organic homemade skincare routine at home is a rewarding and empowering journey that allows you to take control of what you put on your skin. By using natural ingredients, basic tools, and simple recipes, you can create effective skincare products that promote healthy, glowing skin without the use of harsh chemicals or additives. With dedication, creativity, and a commitment to self-care, you can transform your skincare routine into a nourishing and rejuvenating experience that celebrates the beauty of nature and the power of holistic skincare.

Chapter 3

What are organic products:Exploring Organic Skincare Products; Nature's Gift for Radiant Skin.

In recent years, there has been a growing interest in organic skincare products as more people seek natural alternatives to conventional cosmetics. Organic skincare products harness the power of plant-based ingredients, botanical extracts, and natural oils to nourish, protect, and rejuvenate the skin. In this guide, we'll explore what organic skincare products are, their benefits, and how they differ from conventional skincare options.

Understanding Organic Skincare Products:

Organic skincare products are formulations made from ingredients sourced from organic farming practices. These ingredients are grown without the use of synthetic pesticides,herbicides,fertilizers,or genetically modified organisms (GMOs). Additionally, organic skincare products are free from harsh chemicals, artificial fragrances, parabens, sulfates, and other potentially harmful additives commonly found in conventional skincare products.

Key Features of Organic Skincare Products:

1. Natural Ingredients: Organic skincare products are formulated with natural ingredients derived from plants, fruits, flowers, and botanicals. These ingredients are carefully selected for their therapeutic properties and skin-loving benefits, such as hydration, nourishment, and antioxidant protection.

2. Certified Organic: To ensure the authenticity and quality of organic skincare products, look for certifications from reputable organizations such as the Soil Association, Ecocert, or USDA Organic. These certifications guarantee that the ingredients used in the products are grown

and processed according to strict organic standards.

3. Ethical and Sustainable: Organic skincare products are often produced using environmentally sustainable practices that minimize harm to the planet and promote biodiversity. Many organic skincare brands prioritize ethical sourcing, fair trade practices, and eco-friendly packaging to minimize their carbon footprint and support sustainable agriculture.

Benefits of Organic Skincare Products:

1. Gentle and Nourishing: Organic skincare products are formulated with gentle, non-toxic ingredients that are suitable for all skin types, including sensitive and allergy-prone skin. These products help soothe irritation, calm inflammation, and restore the skin's natural balance without causing harm or irritation.

2. Potent Antioxidants: Organic skincare products are rich in antioxidants, vitamins, and minerals that help protect the skin

against environmental damage, pollution, and oxidative stress. Antioxidants help neutralize free radicals and prevent premature aging, leaving the skin looking youthful, radiant, and rejuvenated.

3. Eco-Friendly: Choosing organic skincare products supports sustainable farming practices, reduces the use of harmful chemicals, and minimizes environmental pollution. By opting for organic skincare, you can contribute to a healthier planet and promote biodiversity while caring for your skin.

Difference Between Organic and Conventional Skincare:

Conventional skincare products often contain synthetic chemicals, preservatives, fragrances, and fillers that may be harsh or irritating to the skin. In contrast, organic skincare products use natural, plant-based ingredients that are free from harmful chemicals and additives, making them safer, gentler, and more nourishing for the skin.

Conclusion:

Organic skincare products offer a natural and holistic approach to skincare that promotes health, wellness, and sustainability. By choosing organic skincare, you can nourish your skin with the purest ingredients nature has to offer, while supporting ethical and environmentally friendly practices. Whether you're looking to soothe sensitive skin, combat signs of aging, or simply enhance your natural beauty, organic skincare products provide a safe, effective, and eco-conscious solution for radiant, healthy skin.

Chapter 4

Understanding the Difference Between Organic and Artificial Products

In the realm of skincare, consumers are presented with a myriad of options, from organic formulations boasting natural ingredients to artificial products filled with synthetic compounds. Understanding the difference between organic and artificial skincare products is essential for making informed choices about what we put on our skin. In this guide, we'll delve into the distinctions between these two types of skincare, exploring their ingredients, benefits, and potential impacts on our skin and the environment.

Organic Skincare Products:

Organic skincare products are formulated with ingredients derived from natural sources and produced using organic farming practices. These products prioritize the use of plant-based extracts, botanical oils, and herbal infusions, free from synthetic pesticides, herbicides, fertilizers, and genetically modified organisms (GMOs). Key features of organic skincare include:

1. Natural Ingredients: Organic skincare products harness the power of nature's bounty, utilizing plant-based ingredients rich in vitamins, minerals, antioxidants, and essential fatty acids. These ingredients nourish, hydrate, and protect the skin while promoting a healthy and radiant complexion.

2. Certified Organic: To ensure authenticity and quality, organic skincare products often carry certifications from reputable organizations such as the Soil Association, Ecocert, or USDA Organic. These certifications guarantee that the ingredients used in the products are grown and processed according to strict organic standards.

3. Environmental Sustainability: Organic skincare brands prioritize sustainability and eco-conscious practices, from ethical

sourcing and fair trade partnerships to eco-friendly packaging and minimal environmental impact. By choosing organic skincare, consumers can support regenerative agriculture and reduce their carbon footprint.

Artificial Skincare Products:

Artificial skincare products, also known as conventional or synthetic skincare, are formulated with synthetic compounds, chemicals, preservatives, and fragrances. While these products may offer immediate results, they often contain ingredients that can be harsh, irritating, or harmful to the skin and the environment. Key features of artificial skincare include:

1. Synthetic Ingredients: Artificial skincare products rely on synthetic compounds and laboratory-created ingredients to achieve specific skincare goals, such as anti-aging, acne treatment, or skin brightening. These ingredients may include parabens, sulfates, phthalates, synthetic fragrances, and petroleum-derived compounds.

2. Short-Term Benefits: Artificial skincare products may provide immediate results, such as smoother texture, reduced wrinkles, or clearer complexion. However, long-term use of these products may lead to adverse effects, including skin irritation, allergic reactions, or disruption of the skin's natural barrier function.

3. Environmental Concerns: The production and disposal of artificial skincare products can have negative impacts on the environment, contributing to pollution, water contamination, and habitat destruction. Additionally, the use of synthetic chemicals in skincare formulations may pose risks to aquatic ecosystems and wildlife.

Distinguishing Between Organic and Artificial Skincare:

1. Ingredient Transparency: Organic skincare products prioritize transparency and ingredient integrity, clearly listing natural and organic ingredients on their

labels. In contrast, artificial skincare products may contain complex chemical compositions and proprietary blends that are difficult to decipher.

2. Safety and Efficacy: Organic skincare products are formulated with gentle, non-toxic ingredients that are safe for all skin types, including sensitive and allergy-prone skin. Artificial skincare products may contain harsh chemicals and preservatives that can cause skin irritation, allergic reactions, or long-term damage with prolonged use.

3. Environmental Impact: Organic skincare products support sustainable farming practices, ethical sourcing, and eco-friendly production methods that minimize harm to the environment. Artificial skincare products may contribute to pollution, habitat destruction, and environmental degradation through the use of synthetic chemicals and unsustainable manufacturing processes.

Conclusion:
Understanding the difference between organic and artificial skincare products empowers consumers to make informed choices that prioritize their health, well-being, and the environment. While artificial skincare products may offer short-term benefits, organic skincare provides a natural, holistic approach to skincare that nourishes the skin without compromising on safety, efficacy, or sustainability. By choosing organic skincare, consumers can embrace the transformative power of nature and cultivate a radiant, healthy complexion while supporting ethical and eco-conscious practices.

Chapter 5

Exploring Types of Organic Body Lotions and DIY Recipes

Organic body lotions offer a nourishing and luxurious way to hydrate and pamper your skin while avoiding harsh chemicals and additives. By harnessing the power of natural ingredients, you can create personalized body lotions tailored to your skin's needs. In this guide, we'll explore different types of organic body lotions and provide simple DIY recipes to prepare them at home, allowing you to indulge in the goodness of nature and promote healthy, glowing skin.

1. Moisturizing Body Lotion:
- Ingredients:
  - ½ cup organic shea butter
  - ¼ cup organic coconut oil
  - 2 tablespoons organic jojoba oil

- Optional: a few drops of essential oil for fragrance (e.g., lavender, rose, or citrus)
- **Instructions:**

1. In a double boiler, melt the shea butter and coconut oil over low heat until fully liquefied.

2. Remove from heat and stir in the jojoba oil and essential oil, if using.

3. Allow the mixture to cool slightly before transferring it to a clean, sterilized jar or container.

4. Let the body lotion solidify at room temperature or in the refrigerator until it reaches a creamy consistency.

5. To use, apply a small amount of the lotion to clean, dry skin and massage gently until absorbed.

2. Soothing Body Butter:
- **Ingredients:**
  - ½ cup organic cocoa butter
  - ¼ cup organic shea butter
  - 2 tablespoons organic sweet almond oil

- Optional: a few drops of essential oil for fragrance (e.g., chamomile, calendula, or lavender)

- Instructions:

1. In a heat-safe bowl, combine the cocoa butter and shea butter.

2. Place the bowl over a pot of simmering water (double boiler) and melt the butters together, stirring occasionally until smooth and melted.

3. Remove from heat and stir in the sweet almond oil and essential oil, if desired.

4. Allow the mixture to cool for a few minutes before transferring it to a clean, sterilized jar or container.

5. Let the body butter solidify at room temperature or in the refrigerator until it reaches a creamy consistency.

6. Apply a small amount of the body butter to your skin, focusing on dry or rough areas, and massage gently until absorbed.

3. Refreshing Aloe Vera Body Lotion:
- Ingredients:

- ½ cup organic aloe vera gel
- 2 tablespoons organic coconut oil
- 1 tablespoon organic sweet almond oil
- Optional: a few drops of essential oil for fragrance (e.g., peppermint, eucalyptus, or tea tree)

- Instructions:

1. In a mixing bowl, combine the aloe vera gel, coconut oil, and sweet almond oil.

2. Using a hand mixer or whisk, blend the ingredients together until smooth and well combined.

3. Add the essential oil, if using, and mix again to incorporate.

4. Transfer the body lotion to a clean, sterilized pump bottle or jar for easy dispensing.

5. Store the lotion in the refrigerator for a refreshing, cooling effect, and shake well before each use.

6. Apply the aloe vera body lotion to your skin as needed, massaging gently until absorbed.

Conclusion:

Indulge in the nourishing benefits of organic body lotions by preparing your own homemade formulations using natural, plant-based ingredients. Whether you prefer a rich and moisturizing body butter, a light and soothing lotion, or a refreshing aloe vera gel, there's a DIY recipe to suit your skin's needs and preferences. By embracing the goodness of nature and avoiding harsh chemicals and additives, you can promote healthy, radiant skin and indulge in the luxurious experience of self-care. So why wait? Get creative in the kitchen and treat yourself to the ultimate skincare indulgence with homemade organic body lotions.

Chapter 6

Exploring Types of Organic Face and Body Scrubs and DIY Recipes

Organic face and body scrubs offer a gentle yet effective way to exfoliate and rejuvenate the skin, leaving it soft, smooth, and radiant. By incorporating natural ingredients into your skincare routine, you can create personalized scrubs tailored to your skin's needs. In this guide, we'll explore different types of organic face and body scrubs and provide simple DIY recipes to prepare them at home, allowing you to indulge in the rejuvenating power of nature and achieve a healthy, glowing complexion.

1. Exfoliating Sugar Scrub:

- Ingredients:

  - 1 cup organic brown sugar or white sugar
  - ½ cup organic coconut oil
  - Optional: a few drops of essential oil for fragrance (e.g., lavender, lemon, or peppermint)

- Instructions:

1. In a mixing bowl, combine the sugar and coconut oil.

2. Stir well until the ingredients are evenly mixed and the scrub has a grainy texture.

3. Add the essential oil, if using, and mix again to incorporate.

4. Transfer the sugar scrub to a clean, sterilized jar or container for storage.

5. To use, apply a small amount of the scrub to damp skin and massage gently in circular motions, focusing on areas of dry or rough skin. Rinse thoroughly with warm water and pat dry.

2. Nourishing Coffee Scrub:
- Ingredients:
- ½ cup organic coffee grounds (freshly ground)
- ½ cup organic coconut oil
- Optional: 1 tablespoon organic honey or raw sugar for added hydration and exfoliation
- Instructions:
1. In a mixing bowl, combine the coffee grounds and coconut oil.

2. If desired, add the honey or raw sugar to the mixture for added hydration and exfoliation.

3. Stir well until the ingredients are thoroughly combined and the scrub has a gritty texture.

4. Transfer the coffee scrub to a clean, sterilized jar or container for storage.

5. To use, apply the scrub to damp skin and massage gently in circular motions, paying special attention to areas of cellulite or rough patches. Rinse off with warm water and pat dry.

3. Brightening Turmeric Scrub:
- Ingredients:
  - ½ cup organic brown sugar or white sugar
  - ¼ cup organic coconut oil
  - 1 teaspoon organic turmeric powder
  - Optional: a few drops of lemon essential oil for added brightening effects

- Instructions:

1. In a mixing bowl, combine the sugar, coconut oil, and turmeric powder.

2. Stir well until the ingredients are evenly mixed and the scrub has a vibrant yellow color.

3. Add the lemon essential oil, if using, and mix again to incorporate.

4. Transfer the turmeric scrub to a clean, sterilized jar or container for storage.

5. To use, apply a small amount of the scrub to damp skin and massage gently in circular motions, focusing on areas of dullness or uneven skin tone. Rinse off with warm water and pat dry.

Conclusion:

Indulge in the rejuvenating benefits of organic face and body scrubs by preparing your own homemade formulations using natural, plant-based ingredients. Whether you prefer a gentle sugar scrub, an invigorating coffee scrub, or a brightening turmeric scrub, there's a DIY recipe to suit your skin's needs and preferences. By embracing the goodness of nature and avoiding harsh chemicals and additives, you can promote healthy, glowing skin and indulge in the luxurious experience of self-care. So why wait? Get creative in the kitchen and treat yourself to the ultimate skincare indulgence with homemade organic scrubs.

Chapter 7

Embrace Your Natural Glow: DIY Organic Moisturizers for Fair and Dark Skin Tones

Moisturizing is a vital step in any skincare routine, helping to hydrate, nourish, and protect the skin from environmental stressors. Organic moisturizers offer a gentle yet effective way to achieve healthy, radiant skin without the use of harsh chemicals or additives. In this guide, we'll explore DIY organic moisturizer recipes tailored for both fair and dark skin tones, allowing you to embrace your natural beauty and promote optimal skin health with ingredients found in nature.

Organic Moisturizer for Fair Skin:
Fair skin often requires lightweight, non-comedogenic moisturizers that provide hydration without leaving a greasy or heavy residue. The following DIY recipe features

natural ingredients that nourish and protect delicate fair skin:

Ingredients:

- 2 tablespoons organic aloe vera gel
- 1 tablespoon organic jojoba oil
- 1 teaspoon organic rosehip seed oil
- 5 drops organic lavender essential oil

Instructions:

1. In a small mixing bowl, combine the aloe vera gel, jojoba oil, and rosehip seed oil.

2. Add the lavender essential oil and mix well to ensure all ingredients are evenly incorporated.

3. Transfer the moisturizer to a clean, sterilized jar or container for storage.

4. To use, apply a small amount of the moisturizer to clean, dry skin and massage gently until absorbed.

5. Use daily as part of your morning and evening skincare routine for soft, supple, and hydrated skin.

Organic Moisturizer for Dark Skin:

Dark skin tones often benefit from rich, nourishing moisturizers that help enhance natural radiance and provide long-lasting hydration. The following DIY recipe features luxurious ingredients that deeply moisturize and rejuvenate dark skin:

Ingredients:
- 3 tablespoons organic shea butter
- 2 tablespoons organic coconut oil
- 1 tablespoon organic argan oil
- 5 drops organic frankincense essential oil

Instructions:
1. In a heat-safe bowl, combine the shea butter and coconut oil.
2. Place the bowl over a pot of simmering water (double boiler) and melt the butters together, stirring occasionally until smooth and melted.
3. Remove from heat and stir in the argan oil and frankincense essential oil.
4. Allow the mixture to cool for a few minutes before transferring it to a clean, sterilized jar or container for storage.

5. Let the moisturizer solidify at room temperature or in the refrigerator until it reaches a creamy consistency.

6. To use, apply a small amount of the moisturizer to clean, dry skin and massage gently until absorbed.

7. Use daily as part of your morning and evening skincare routine for nourished, glowing, and radiant skin.

Conclusion:

Achieving healthy, radiant skin is achievable for individuals of all skin tones with the right skincare regimen. By preparing your own organic moisturizers at home using natural, plant-based ingredients, you can nourish and protect your skin while embracing your unique complexion. Whether you have fair or dark skin, these DIY moisturizer recipes offer a luxurious and effective way to promote optimal skin health and enhance your natural beauty. So why wait? Embrace your natural glow and indulge in the goodness of organic skincare with homemade moisturizers tailored to your skin's needs.

Chapter 8

Unveiling the Power of Vitamin C Serum: Benefits and DIY Organic Recipes

Vitamin C serum has gained popularity in the skincare world for its potent antioxidant properties and ability to brighten, firm, and protect the skin from environmental damage. While commercial vitamin C serums are readily available, preparing your own organic version at home allows you to customize the formulation and ensure the use of natural, skin-loving ingredients. In this guide, we'll explore the benefits of vitamin C serum and provide simple DIY organic recipes to prepare it at home, helping you achieve healthy, radiant skin naturally.

Understanding Vitamin C Serum:

Vitamin C serum is a skincare product formulated with a high concentration of vitamin C, also known as ascorbic acid. This powerful antioxidant helps neutralize free radicals, stimulate collagen production, and brighten the complexion, resulting in firmer, smoother, and more youthful-looking skin. Vitamin C serum is suitable for all skin types and can address various skincare concerns, including dullness, uneven skin tone, fine lines, and sun damage.

Benefits of Vitamin C Serum:

1. Antioxidant Protection: Vitamin C serum helps protect the skin from oxidative stress and environmental aggressors, such as UV radiation, pollution, and free radicals, which can lead to premature aging and skin damage.

2. Collagen Synthesis: Vitamin C stimulates collagen production in the skin, promoting elasticity, firmness, and resilience, while

reducing the appearance of fine lines, wrinkles, and sagging.

3. Brightening Effect: Vitamin C inhibits melanin production and reduces hyperpigmentation, age spots, and sun damage, resulting in a brighter, more even-toned complexion.

4. Healing Properties: Vitamin C has anti-inflammatory and wound-healing properties, making it effective for soothing redness, irritation, and acne breakouts, while promoting skin repair and regeneration.

DIY Organic Vitamin C Serum Recipes:

1. Simple Vitamin C Serum:
- Ingredients:
  - 1 teaspoon organic vitamin C powder (ascorbic acid)
  - 1 tablespoon organic vegetable glycerin or aloe vera gel

- 2 tablespoons distilled water or organic rose water

- Instructions:

1. In a small glass bottle or dropper, combine the vitamin C powder and vegetable glycerin or aloe vera gel.

2. Stir or shake well until the vitamin C powder is fully dissolved and the mixture is smooth.

3. Add the distilled water or rose water to the mixture and shake again to combine.

4. Store the serum in a cool, dark place away from direct sunlight to maintain its potency.

5. To use, apply a few drops of the serum to clean, dry skin and gently massage until absorbed. Follow with moisturizer and sunscreen during the day.

2. Hydrating Vitamin C Serum:

- Ingredients:

- 1 teaspoon organic vitamin C powder (ascorbic acid)

- 1 tablespoon organic rosehip seed oil or argan oil

- 1 tablespoon organic vegetable glycerin or honey
- Instructions:

1. In a small glass bottle or dropper, combine the vitamin C powder and rosehip seed oil or argan oil.

2. Stir or shake well until the vitamin C powder is fully dissolved and the mixture is smooth.

3. Add the vegetable glycerin or honey to the mixture and shake again to combine.

4. Store the serum in a cool, dark place away from direct sunlight to maintain its potency.

5. To use, apply a few drops of the serum to clean, dry skin and gently massage until absorbed. Follow with moisturizer or facial oil for added hydration.

Conclusion:

Vitamin C serum is a versatile and effective skincare product that can help improve the overall health and appearance of your skin. By preparing your own organic vitamin C serum at home using natural, skin-loving ingredients, you can harness the power of this potent antioxidant while avoiding harsh chemicals and additives. Whether you're looking to brighten, firm, or protect your skin, these DIY recipes offer a simple and affordable way to incorporate vitamin C into your skincare routine and achieve healthy, radiant skin naturally. So why wait? Unveil the power of vitamin C serum and experience the transformative benefits for yourself.

Chapter 9

Rejuvenate Naturally: DIY Organic Salt and Turmeric Scrub for Glowing Skin

Organic salt and turmeric scrub is a rejuvenating skincare treatment that exfoliates, brightens, and revitalizes the skin, leaving it soft, smooth, and radiant. By harnessing the power of natural ingredients such as salt, turmeric, and nourishing oils, you can create a luxurious scrub that promotes optimal skin health and enhances your natural beauty. In this guide, we'll explore the benefits of organic salt and turmeric scrub and provide a simple DIY recipe to prepare it at home, allowing you to indulge in a spa-like experience and achieve glowing skin naturally.

Benefits of Salt and Turmeric Scrub:
1. Exfoliation: Salt granules gently exfoliate the skin, removing dead skin cells, dirt, and

impurities, while promoting cell turnover and revealing a brighter complexion.

2. Brightening Effect: Turmeric contains curcumin, a natural compound that helps reduce hyperpigmentation, dark spots, and uneven skin tone, resulting in a more radiant and even complexion.

3. Antioxidant Protection: Turmeric and salt are both rich in antioxidants that help neutralize free radicals, protect the skin from environmental damage, and prevent premature aging.

4. Skin Nourishment: Organic oils such as coconut oil or olive oil provide deep hydration, nourishment, and moisture to the skin, leaving it soft, supple, and rejuvenated.

DIY Organic Salt and Turmeric Scrub Recipe:

Ingredients:

- ½ cup organic sea salt or Himalayan pink salt (finely ground)
- 1 tablespoon organic turmeric powder

- 2-3 tablespoons organic coconut oil or olive oil
- Optional: a few drops of essential oil for fragrance (e.g., lavender, rosemary, or citrus)

Instructions:

1. In a mixing bowl, combine the salt and turmeric powder.

2. Gradually add the coconut oil or olive oil to the mixture, stirring well until the ingredients are evenly distributed and the scrub has a wet sand-like consistency. Adjust the amount of oil as needed to achieve your desired texture.

3. If desired, add a few drops of essential oil for fragrance and additional skincare benefits. Stir to incorporate.

4. Transfer the scrub to a clean, sterilized jar or container for storage.

5. To use, dampen your skin with warm water and apply a small amount of the scrub to the desired areas, such as the face, body, or hands.

6. Gently massage the scrub into your skin using circular motions, focusing on areas of dryness, roughness, or uneven texture.

7. Rinse thoroughly with warm water and pat dry. Follow with your favorite moisturizer or body oil for added hydration.

Tips:

- Perform a patch test before using the scrub to check for any allergic reactions or sensitivities, especially if you have sensitive skin.

- Use the scrub 2-3 times per week for best results, avoiding over-exfoliation, which can irritate the skin.

- Store the scrub in a cool, dry place away from direct sunlight to maintain its freshness and potency.

Conclusion:

Organic salt and turmeric scrub is a natural and effective skincare treatment that promotes healthy, glowing skin. By preparing your own DIY scrub at home using simple, organic ingredients, you can enjoy the benefits of exfoliation, brightening, and nourishment without the use of harsh chemicals or additives. Incorporate this luxurious scrub into your skincare routine to rejuvenate your skin and enhance your natural beauty, leaving you with a radiant and luminous complexion. So why wait? Treat yourself to a spa-like experience and indulge in the rejuvenating power of organic salt and turmeric scrub for glowing skin.

Chapter 10

DIY Organic Lip Scrub and Lip Balm: Nourish and Pamper Your Lips Naturally

Organic lip scrub and lip balm are essential components of a healthy lip care routine, providing exfoliation, hydration, and protection for soft, smooth, and kissable lips. By using natural ingredients such as sugar, coconut oil, and beeswax, you can create luxurious lip treatments at home that are free from harsh chemicals and additives. In this guide, we'll explore the benefits of organic lip scrub and lip balm and provide simple DIY recipes to prepare them, allowing you to indulge in self-care and nourish your lips naturally.

Benefits of Lip Scrub and Lip Balm:
1. Exfoliation: Lip scrub helps remove dead skin cells, flakiness, and impurities from the

lips, revealing softer, smoother, and more supple skin underneath.

2. Hydration: Lip balm provides deep hydration and moisture to the lips, preventing dryness, chapping, and cracking, especially in harsh weather conditions.

3. Protection: Lip balm creates a protective barrier on the lips, shielding them from environmental stressors such as wind, sun, and cold temperatures, while locking in moisture and preventing moisture loss.

4. Nourishment: Organic ingredients such as coconut oil, shea butter, and beeswax nourish and replenish the lips with essential vitamins, minerals, and fatty acids, promoting optimal lip health and vitality.

DIY Organic Lip Scrub Recipe:
Ingredients:
- 1 tablespoon organic coconut oil
- 1 tablespoon organic brown sugar or white sugar

- Optional: a few drops of organic honey or vanilla extract for added hydration and fragrance

Instructions:

1. In a small mixing bowl, combine the coconut oil and sugar.

2. If desired, add the honey or vanilla extract to the mixture for added hydration and fragrance.

3. Stir well until all the ingredients are evenly mixed and the scrub has a thick, grainy texture.

4. Transfer the lip scrub to a clean, sterilized jar or container for storage.

5. To use, apply a small amount of the scrub to your lips and gently massage in circular motions for 1-2 minutes.

6. Rinse off with warm water and pat dry. Follow with lip balm for added hydration and protection.

DIY Organic Lip Balm Recipe:
Ingredients:

- 1 tablespoon organic coconut oil

- 1 tablespoon organic beeswax pellets or grated beeswax
- 1 tablespoon organic shea butter or cocoa butter
- Optional: a few drops of organic essential oil for fragrance (e.g., peppermint, lavender, or citrus)

Instructions:

1. In a heat-safe bowl, combine the coconut oil, beeswax, and shea butter.

2. Place the bowl over a pot of simmering water (double boiler) and heat gently until the ingredients are fully melted, stirring occasionally.

3. Once melted, remove from heat and add the essential oil, if using. Stir well to incorporate.

4. Carefully pour the mixture into clean, sterilized lip balm containers or tubes.

5. Allow the lip balm to cool and solidify at room temperature or in the refrigerator for 1-2 hours.

6. Once solidified, cap the lip balm containers or tubes and store them in a cool, dry place away from direct sunlight.

7. To use, apply the lip balm to your lips as needed throughout the day for hydration, nourishment, and protection.

Conclusion:

Organic lip scrub and lip balm are simple yet effective skincare treatments that promote healthy, hydrated, and beautiful lips. By preparing your own DIY lip care products at home using natural, organic ingredients, you can indulge in self-care and pamper your lips with luxurious treatments that are free from harsh chemicals and additives. Incorporate these homemade lip scrub and lip balm into your daily skincare routine to nourish, protect, and enhance the natural beauty of your lips. So why wait? Treat yourself to the ultimate lip care experience and enjoy soft, smooth, and kissable lips all year round.

Chapter 11

The Essential Do's and Don'ts of Organic Skincare Routine

Embracing an organic skincare routine offers numerous benefits for your skin and overall well-being. However, it's important to understand the best practices and avoid common pitfalls to achieve optimal results while using organic skincare products. In this guide, we'll explore the essential do's and don'ts of an organic skincare routine, helping you to nourish and care for your skin effectively while prioritizing natural ingredients and sustainable practices.

The Do's of Organic Skincare Routine:

1. Do Choose High-Quality Organic Products: Opt for organic skincare products made from high-quality, natural ingredients sourced from organic farming practices. Look for certifications from reputable

organizations to ensure authenticity and purity.

2. Do Patch Test New Products: Before incorporating new organic skincare products into your routine, perform a patch test on a small area of your skin to check for any allergic reactions or sensitivities.

3. Do Cleanse and Moisturize Daily: Cleanse your skin twice daily using a gentle, organic cleanser to remove dirt, oil, and impurities. Follow up with a nourishing organic moisturizer to hydrate and protect your skin from environmental stressors.

4. Do Exfoliate Regularly: Incorporate exfoliation into your skincare routine 1-2 times per week to remove dead skin cells and promote cell turnover. Choose a gentle organic exfoliant to avoid irritation and over-exfoliation.

5. Do Protect Your Skin from Sun Damage: Apply a broad-spectrum organic sunscreen with SPF 30 or higher daily to protect your skin from harmful UV rays and prevent premature aging, sunburns, and skin cancer.

6. Do Practice Patience and Consistency: Give your organic skincare routine time to work and be consistent with your regimen. Results may take time to appear, so stick to your routine and be patient with your skin's natural healing process.

The Don'ts of Organic Skincare Routine:

1. Don't Overload Your Skin with Products: Avoid using too many skincare products at once, as this can overwhelm your skin and disrupt its natural balance. Stick to a simple, minimalist routine with a few key products that address your skin's specific needs.

2. Don't Ignore Ingredient Labels: Always read the ingredient labels of organic skincare products carefully to avoid potentially harmful additives, fragrances, and synthetic chemicals. Look for familiar, natural ingredients that are safe and beneficial for your skin.

3. Don't Skip Patch Testing: Never skip the patch test step when trying new organic skincare products, even if they claim to be gentle or suitable for sensitive skin. Patch testing helps prevent adverse reactions and ensures product compatibility with your skin.

4. Don't Over-Exfoliate: Avoid over-exfoliating your skin, as this can lead to irritation, redness, and sensitivity. Limit exfoliation to 1-2 times per week and choose gentle organic exfoliants that are suitable for your skin type.

5. Don't Forget Sun Protection: Don't neglect sun protection, even on cloudy or overcast days. UV rays can penetrate through clouds and cause sun damage, so always wear sunscreen as part of your daily skincare routine.

6. Don't Disregard Your Skin's Needs: Listen to your skin and adjust your skincare routine as needed based on changes in your skin's condition, environment, and lifestyle. Pay attention to any signs of irritation,

dryness, or sensitivity, and modify your routine accordingly.

Conclusion:

Following the do's and don'ts of an organic skincare routine is essential for achieving healthy, radiant skin while prioritizing natural ingredients and sustainable practices. By choosing high-quality organic products, cleansing, moisturizing, and protecting your skin daily, and avoiding common pitfalls such as over-exfoliation and neglecting sun protection, you can nurture your skin's natural beauty and support its overall health and well-being. So embrace an organic skincare routine, be mindful of what you apply to your skin, and enjoy the transformative benefits of natural skincare.